Paleo Dump Dinners:

30 Paleo Dump Dinner Recipes your Kids will Love

Henry Brooke

Table of Contents

Introduction

Welcome to the Paleo Dump Dinners recipe and cookbook, we would like to start off by saying thank you for choosing us and trying what we have to offer to our amazing consumers such as yourself and your delightful kids. Each and every single one of the recipes is made to be delicious as well as nutritious. This is simply because that they are all jam-packed with the vitamins, minerals, and nutrients that are essential to the body in order for it function properly.

We encourage you to try all of the recipes at least once and then we hope that our recipes have inspired you to make recipes and variations of our meals of your own. If you do make something of your own, please send us the recipe for us to try; we would love to see what it tastes like. Some of the recipes within this cookbook may take longer than others to make but that is based on the kinds of ingredients used as well as the amount of ingredients used. A few other factors may be the temperature you cook it at based on when you are planning to actually eat and how often you check it, stir it or even add to it.

Examples of what some paleo dump dinners can be are sweet potato soup, fish fry, a chicken satay, and Italian chicken salad and much, much more. There are even all kinds of unique and tasty bread recipes that you can make in which are paleo dump recipes; there are breads for dinners and dessert breads, all of which can be in as little as five minutes total. When it comes to the recipes such as the ones in this cookbook it comes down to finding and combining the flavors that work best with each other; the ones that work together are the best ones to use. For instance, some of the more popular paleo dump flavor combinations are zucchini and walnuts that are chopped, carrots with some pumpkin spice, apples and cinnamon or apples with cranberries, and tons more. Some of these combinations or others that you may find may not sound appealing but they taste really good. Remember that you should not judge a book by the cover so don't say that you don't like something if you have never even tried it beforehand. With that being said thanks to the paleo dump dinners you can now make whatever it is that you craving for because you can be sure to find a combination that does just what you are looking for.

Enjoy making these meals as well as eating them with your family; you will love it and so will your kids. These recipes are hands down all crowd pleasers and you won't be disappointed with them; make them as is or to your tasting. There is a lot you can do when it comes to dump dinners; they may be easy to make but the combining of the right ingredients is what makes it so good and just like an art form.

Thai Chicken Curry
Serves: 4

Ingredients:
4 chicken thighs
1 teaspoon red curry powder
1 teaspoon red curry paste
14 ounce coconut milk
1 cup snap peas
2 tablespoons peanut butter
½ sweet onion (chopped)
½ cup cilantro (chopped)
1 teaspoon basil (dried)
½ red bell pepper (chopped)
2 tablespoons liquid amino acid
1/8 teaspoon red pepper flakes
½ teaspoon brown sugar

Directions:
1. In a crock pot add the spices followed by the vegetables. Stir.
2. Next add the chicken and allow it to cook on high heat for approximately 3 hours.
3. Serve!

Nutritional Information:
Calories: 434 kcal, Fats: 34.9grams, Carbohydrates: 11.9 grams, Protein: 22.2 grams

Quick Chicken
Serves 4-5

Ingredients:
1 lb. chicken
¼ cup water
½ cup brown sugar
½ cup Paleo Ketchup
3-4 tbsp onion soup mix (dry)

Directions:
1. Place all the ingredients in a baking dish.
2. Bake at 350 degrees for approximately an hour.
3. Serve!

Serves: 4

Ingredients:
4 chicken thighs (trimmed)
1 cup all purpose flour
1 cup pineapple chunks
¾ cup fresh pineapple juice
2 tablespoons Paleo ketchup
½ cup coconut aminos
1/3 cup brown sugar
1 garlic clove (minced)

Directions:
1. Place the chicken in the crock pot and top it off with pineapple.
2. In a mixing bowl, whisk together the rest of the ingredients. Now add this mixture to your crock pot
3. Cook on low heat for approximately four hours.

Nutritional Information:
Calories: 448 kcal, Fats: 11.7grams, Carbohydrates: 62.2grams, Protein: 23.6 grams

Beef Vegetable Stew
Serves: 4

Ingredients:
2 lbs. grass-fed beef (organic; cubed)
4 cups beef broth (organic)
3 potatoes (peeled; sliced)
2 carrots (peeled; sliced)
2 celery stalks (sliced)
5 garlic cloves (chopped)
1 cup onions (trimmed; peeled)
1 cup red wine (dry)
2 teaspoons Italian herbs (dried)
1 bay leaf
2 tablespoons olive oil (extra virgin)
Sea salt (to taste)
Ground pepper (to taste)

Directions:
1. In a shallow dish marinade the beef with salt. Set aside.
2. In a crock pot, place the beef cubes along with olive oil over medium high heat.
5. Now add the vegetables along rest of the ingredients.
6. Cover and cook for approximately 4 to 5 hours on high heat.
7. Serve!

Nutritional Information:
Calories: 321, Fats: 22.8 g, Carbohydrates: 17.1 g, Protein: 34g

Mexican Chuck Roast
Serves: 12

Ingredients:
4 pounds chuck roast
1 onion (chopped)
1 cup green chili pepper (diced)
5 ounce hot pepper sauce
1 teaspoon ground black pepper
1 teaspoon salt
1 teaspoon chili powder
1 teaspoon garlic powder
1 teaspoon cayenne pepper
2 tablespoons canola oil

Directions:
1. Start by seasoning the roast with salt and pepper.
2. Place the roast along with the rest of the ingredients in your crock pot
3. Add water so that it covers one third of the roast.
4. Cook on high heat for approximately 6 hours and then reduce the heat to low and continue cooking for another 3 to 4 hours.
5. Serve

Nutritional Information:
Calories: 260 kcal, Fats: 19.1grams, Carbohydrates: 3.3grams, Protein: 18.4 grams

Cranberry Pork

Serves: 6

Ingredients:
3 pound pork loin roast (boneless)
16 ounce cranberry sauce
1 onion (sliced)
1 cup salad dressing (French)

Directions:
1. Place the pork loin in the crock pot and top it off with the rest of the ingredients.
2. Allow the pork to cook on high heat for approximately 4 hours.
3. Serve!

Nutritional Information:
Calories: 374 kcal, Fats: 15.1grams, Carbohydrates: 32.9grams, Protein: 26.8 grams

Zesty Chicken
Serves 4

Ingredients:
1 lb chicken
3 tbsp lemon juice
3 garlic cloves (minced)
4 tbsp olive oil
2 tbsp parsley (chopped)
¼ tsp ground pepper
2 tbsp grass fed butter

Directions:
1. Place all the ingredients in a baking dish.
2. Bake at 350 degrees for approximately an hour.
3. Serve!

Dump Steak with Mashed Potatoes
Serve 4-5

Ingredients:
1 lb steak
15 ounce tomatoes (diced; canned)
2 ounce beef and onion soup mix (dry)
2 ounce brown gravy mix (dry)

Directions:
1. Combine all the ingredients in a zip lock bag and freeze over night.
2. Thaw and bake at 350 degrees F for approximately 2 hours.
3. Serve over mashed potatoes.

Cantonese Chicken
Serves 4

Ingredients:
1 lb chicken (cubed)
¼ cup honey
¼ cup coconut aminos
½ cup ketchup
2 tbsp lemon juice
Cilantro (for garnishing)

Directions:
1. Place all the ingredients in a baking dish.
2. Bake at 350 degrees for approximately an hour.
3. Garnish it with cilantro and serve!

Nutritional Information:
Calories: 386 kcal, Fats: 9grams, Carbohydrates: 12grams, Protein: 28grams

Thanksgiving Style Turkey Legs
Serves: 6

Ingredients:
6 turkey legs (washed)
Salt and pepper (to taste)
3 teaspoons poultry seasoning

Directions:
1. Place the turkey legs in a crock pot.
2. Now dump all the seasoning on top.
3. Allow it to cook for approximately 7 to 8 hours over low heat.
4. Serve!

Nutritional Information:
Calories: 217 kcal, Fats: 6.9grams, Carbohydrates: 0.2grams, Protein: 36.3 grams

Orange Chicken

Serves: 4

Ingredients:
1 pound chicken breast (boneless, halved)
12 ounce orange flavored beverage
½ cup coconut aminos

Directions:
1. Place the chicken breasts in the crock pot. Top it off with the rest of the ingredients.
2. Allow the chicken to cook on low heat for approximately five to six hours.
3. Serve with brown rice.

Nutritional Information:
Calories: 357 kcal, Fats: 2.7grams, Carbohydrates: 053grams, Protein: 27.8 grams

Beef Chili
Serves: 6

Ingredients:
1 lb. ground beef (browned and drained)
14 oz. beef broth
1 cup chopped onion
3 stalks of celery
2 garlic cloves (minced)
1 can tomato sauce
1 can tomatoes (with juice)
1 cup water
2teaspoon chili powder
½ teaspoon cumin
½ teaspoon paprika
½ teaspoon oregano
1 teaspoon salt
1 teaspoon black pepper
A dash of cayenne pepper

Directions:
1. Place a crock pot over low heat.
2. Add all the ingredients to it. Cover and allow it to cook for approximately six to eight hours over low heat.

Nutritional Information:
Calories: 59; Fat: 9 g; Protein: 4.4g; Carbohydrates: 1.6g

Squash Quinoa Casserole

Serves: one casserole

Ingredients:
12 ounces tomatillos (chopped)
1 pint cherry tomatoes (chopped)
1 bell pepper (chopped)
½ cup onion (chopped)
1 tablespoon lime juice
1 teaspoon sea salt
1 cup of quinoa
1 cup of paneer
2 lbs yellow squash (sliced)
2 tablespoons of oregano

Directions:
1. Place everything in the crock pot and cook on low for four hours.
2. Serve and enjoy.

Nutritional Information:
Calories: 111 kcal, Fats: 3 grams, Carbohydrates: 18 grams, Protein: 5 grams

Turkey stew with green chilies
Serves: 5

Ingredients:
1 ½ cups butternut squash (peeled and diced)
1 lb. ground turkey
2 potatoes (peeled and diced)
3 carrots (peeled and chopped)
1 onion (diced)
4 cloves garlic (minced)
1 teaspoon cumin
1 teaspoon chili powder
1 cup roasted chopped green chili
1 quart chicken stock
Sea salt and black pepper to taste
2 teaspoons agave nectar, as needed

Directions:
1. Add the turkey to the slow cooker along with the remaining ingredients. Stir well to combine.
2. Cover and cook until the pork is done.
3. Serve

Nutritional information:
Calories: 423 kcal; Fats: 13.5g; Carbohydrates: 44.7g; Protein: 36.3g

Spicy Spinach Sauce
Serves: 4

Ingredients:
2 cans tomatoes (peeled and crushed)
10 ounce spinach (frozen, chopped, thawed and drained)
1 onion (chopped)
1/3 cup carrot (grated)
2 ½ tablespoons red pepper (crushed)
5 garlic cloves (minced)
1 can tomato paste
1 can mushrooms (sliced and drained)
2 tablespoons dried oregano
2 tablespoons sea salt
2 tablespoons dried basil
2 bay leaves
¼ cup olive oil (extra virgin)

Directions:
1. Dump the spinach with the rest of the ingredients in a crock pot.
2. Cover and cook for approximately 5 hours over high heat.
3. Serve.

Nutritional Information:
Calories; 176, Fats 8.2g, Carbohydrates 25.1g, Protein 6.6g

Caribbean Chicken
Serves 4-6

Ingredients:
6-7 pieces chicken breasts
¼ cup brown sugar
1 can pineapple (chunks with juice)
½ tsp nutmeg
½ cup raisins
1/3 cup orange juice

Directions
1. Place all the ingredients in a baking dish.
2. Bake at 350 degrees for approximately 60 minutes
3. Serve!

Pollo Pibil
Serves: 8

Ingredients:
3 lbs. chicken thighs (boneless)
2 habaneros (seeded and diced)
¼ cup chicken broth
4 tablespoons achiote paste
½ cup orange juice
½ cup apple cider vinegar
1 onion (chopped)
1 teaspoon coriander
1 teaspoon cumin
1 teaspoon oregano (dried)
3 garlic cloves (diced)
Salt and pepper (to taste)

Directions:
1. Place all the ingredients into your slow cooker.
2. Cover and cook for at least four hours or until the chicken can be easily shredded.
3. Serve!

Nutritional Information:
Calories: 139.8; Fat: 4.1 g; Protein: 20.8g; Carbohydrates: 3.8g

Bacon and Spinach Quiche
Serves: 8

Ingredients:
10 eggs (beaten)
10 bacon slices (chopped)
½ cup spinach (chopped)
1 cup agave nectar
1 tablespoon grass fed butter
8 oz. paneer (shredded)
½ teaspoon black pepper

Directions:
1. Add all the ingredients into your slow cooker.
2. Allow it to cook on low heat for approximately 4 hours.
3. Serve!

Nutritional Information:
Calories: 346 kcal; Fat: 28.5g; Carbohydrates: 2.2g; Protein: 21.2g

Beef Stroganoff
Serves 6-8

Ingredients:
2 lbs stew meat (sliced)
1 package onion soup mix
1 can Ginger Ale
1 cup mushrooms (sliced)
2 tbsp corn starch
1 can cream of mushroom soup

Directions:
1. Place all the ingredients into your crock pot.
2. Cook on low heat for approximately 6-7 hours.
3. Serve!

Rabbit Stew
Serves: 6

Ingredients:
3oz. rabbit (cut into pieces)
½ lb. pork belly (smoked, cubes)
2 cups white wine (dry)
2 tablespoons grass fed butter
1 sprig rosemary
2 bay leaves
1 onion (large; thinly sliced)
2 tablespoons sea salt
1 teaspoon whole peppercorn

Directions:
1. Place all the ingredients into your slow cooker.
2. Cover and cook for at least five to six hours.
3. Serve!

Nutritional Information:
Calories: 517; Fat: 32 g; Protein: 36g; Carbohydrates: 2g

Balsamic Chicken

Serves: 6

Ingredients:
4 chicken breasts (boneless; halved, seasoned with salt and pepper)
½ cup balsamic vinegar
2 cans tomatoes (crushed)
1 onion (sliced)
4 garlic cloves
1 teaspoon rosemary (dried)
½ teaspoon thyme (dried)
1 teaspoon oregano (dried)
1 teaspoon basil (dried)
2 tablespoons olive oil (extra virgin)
Salt and pepper (to taste)

Directions:
1. Place all the ingredients in a crock pot.
2. Cook on high heat for approximately four hours or until the juices run clear.
3. Serve!

Nutritional Information:
Calories: 200; Fat: 6.8 g; Protein: 18.6g; Carbohydrates: 17.6g

Serves: 8

Ingredients:
2 lbs. ground pork (precooked)
8 slices of bacon (cooked)
1 medium onion (yellow) (chopped)
3 small green peppers (chopped)
6 oz. tomato paste
1 pack of chili seasoning
1 can of diced tomatoes (drained)
1 teaspoon garlic powder
1 teaspoon onion powder
A dash of cayenne pepper
Salt and pepper (to taste)

Directions:
1. Place all the ingredients in your slow cooker.
2. Cook for approximately six hours on low heat.
3. Serve!

Nutritional Information:
Calories: 492; Fat: 35 g; Protein: 31g; Carbohydrates: 13g

Beef Casserole
Serves 5

Ingredients:
1 lb ground beef (precooked)
2 tbsp grass fed butter
½ cup onion (chopped)
2 cups noodles (uncooked)
1 can tomato sauce
3 cups water
2 tsp coconut aminos
1 tsp sea salt
½ tsp ground pepper
1 cup paneer
½ tsp chili powder

Directions:
1. Preheat the oven to 350 degrees F.
2. Dump in all the ingredients into a ziplock bag and mix together.
3. Spoon into a baking pan and allow it to cook for approximately 45-50 minutes.
4. Serve!

Cashew Chicken

Serves: 6

Ingredients:
2 lbs. chicken thigh
1 bunch scallions (chopped)
1 lb. cashews (raw)
½ onion (white; chopped)
3 tablespoons fish sauce
2 tablespoons agave nectar
3 tablespoons coconut aminos
6 garlic cloves (minced)
¼ teaspoon white pepper
Water

Directions:
1. Place all the ingredients in a crock pot.
2. Cook on high heat for approximately five hours.
3. Sprinkle the cashews on top and serve!

Nutritional Information:
Calories: 651; Fat: 46.4 g; Protein: 30.6g; Carbohydrates: 34.1g

Pumpkin Goulash

Serves: 6

Ingredients:
6 diced tomatoes
1 tablespoon of brown sugar
2 tablespoons of olive oil
1 onion, chopped
1 teaspoon of ginger
1 teaspoon of cinnamon
1 teaspoon of cumin
1 tablespoon of coriander
1 can of garbanzo beans
3 pounds of fresh pumpkin, peeled and cut into small chunks
1 teaspoon of salt
1 teaspoon of cornstarch
¼ cup of water

Directions:
1. Peel and cut the pumpkin up.
2. Chop up everything else that needs to get cut up.
3. Place it all in the slow cooker.
4. Cook on high heat for about four hours.
5. Serve and enjoy!

Nutritional Information:
Calories: 330 kcal, Fats: 7.9 grams, Carbohydrates: 37.2 grams, Protein: 28.4 grams

Butter Chicken
Serves 4-5

Ingredients:
5-6 chicken breasts
3 tbsp peanut butter
1 tbsp coconut aminos
2 tbsp grass fed butter
3 tbsp Paleo Ketchup

Directions:
1. Place all the ingredients in a baking dish.
2. Bake in the oven for approximately an hour at 350 degrees F.
3. Serve with veggies!

Eggplant Sauce
Serves: 2

Ingredients:
1 eggplant
2 14.5-oz. cans diced tomatoes
6 oz. tomato paste (canned)
1 4-oz. can sliced mushrooms; drained
¼ cup red wine (dry)
¼ cup water
½ cup onion (chopped)
2 cloves of garlic (chopped)
1½ teaspoon oregano
1/3 cup olives (pitted)
2 tablespoons fresh parsley; chopped
Vegan cheese (shredded; optional)

Directions:
1. Peel eggplant and cut into small cubes.
2. In the slow cooker combine the eggplant, onion, canned tomatoes with juice, tomato paste, mushrooms, wine, water, garlic, and oregano.
3. Cover the slow cooker and allow it to cook on low heat for approximately 7 to 8 hours.
4. Add the olives and parsley.
5. Serve over cooked rice and sprinkle with vegan cheese.

Nutritional Information:
Calories; 346, Fats 4g, Carbohydrates 65g, Protein 13g

Slow Cooker Mediterranean Stew

Serves: 10

Ingredients:
1 butternut squash - peeled, seeded, and cubed
2 cups eggplant, cubed
2 cups zucchini, cubed
1 (10 ounce) package frozen okra, thawed
1 can tomato sauce
1 cup chopped onion
1 ripe tomato, chopped
1 carrot, sliced
1/2 cup vegetable broth
1/3 cup raisins
1 clove garlic, chopped
1/2 teaspoon ground cumin
1/2 teaspoon ground turmeric
1/4 teaspoon crushed red pepper
1/4 teaspoon ground cinnamon
1/4 teaspoon paprika

Directions:
1. Combine all ingredients together in a slow cooker.
2. Cook on low for approximately 9 hours or until the vegetables have reached your desired tenderness.
3. Serve and enjoy!

Nutritional Information:
Calories: 122 kcal, Fats: 0.5 grams, Carbohydrates: 30.5 grams, Protein: 3.4 grams

Chicken and Broccoli Casserole
Serves: 4

Ingredients:
1 pound broccoli (frozen)
1 pound boiled chicken (cut into chunks)
1 cup chicken broth
½ tablespoon cream
½ pound paneer

Directions:
1. Place all the ingredients in a slow cooker and allow it to cook for approximately 3 to 4 hours on low heat.
2. Serve hot!

Nutritional Information:
Calories: 405, Fats: 46.8 g, Carbohydrates: 15.2 g, Protein: 56.2g

Chicken Soup
Serves 4

Ingredients:
4 chicken breasts
6-7 garlic cloves, chopped
Sea salt (to taste)
Ground pepper (to taste)
2 cups cabbage (shredded)
1 bell pepper (green, deseeded, diced)
1 squash (yellow, diced)
2 zucchini (sliced)
6 potatoes (sliced)
1 4-oz. can green chilies (chopped)
2 tsp sage
2 tsp each of: dried basil, oregano, and parsley
1 can diced tomatoes
2 cups chicken broth
2 tsp grass fed butter

Directions:
1. Dump all the ingredients into your crock pot.
2. Cover the pot and let it cook for up to 5 to 6 hours, or until the chicken is tender and easily breaks apart into pieces.
3. Serve!

Nutritional Information:
Calories: 277 kcal; Fats: 8.9g; Carbohydrates: 13.6g; Protein: 35.0g

Conclusion

We are so sorry that you are now at the end of this recipe book but don't worry because there are a lot of other places that you can turn to for more forms of inspiration and other ideas. Never have to worry about what is for dinner again or how in the world are going to have time to cook dinner and still do everything else. These meals are meant to help save you money, stress and time. It is best to use fresh ingredients for these meals because they take longer to cook and the taste of the meal overall is a lot more refreshing and satisfying because it is so fresh in the first place versus being from a can which is good for a meal that is done in a quicker amount of time.

We hope that you enjoyed reading all of the information that we provided you and also hope that you really liked trying all the recipes. Keep in mind that they are all kid friendly and were created with kids in mind so they are going to surely love it. These recipes are great for anyone of any age; a delicious and warm meal that is homemade is the fastest way to a happy and healthy stomach amongst other things. So easy to make with a very little amount of effort to almost no effort at all to make them, and they come out so great; all you need to do is to have some patience and let time be on your side. You and your kids will thank you.

Trying new things is not scary, it is not hard and it is not disgusting; most certainly it is not a sign of weakness. Trying things that are new is easy, they are fun and meant to show you how to properly experience and live life. To try something new no matter how small or large it may seem, takes courage and is a sign of strength. Help your little one grow up to be tall and strong with great foods from all over and an open mind.

Preview Of 'Ketogenic Diet Rapid Weight Loss Guide: Lose Up To 30 Lbs. In 30 Days'

Want to lose 30 pounds in 30 days?

YOU CAN with the metabolism boosting Ketogenic Diet Plan!

Crash dieting is something pretty much everyone on the planet has tried at one time or another.

NEWSFLASH - It doesn't work!

Livestrong experts report up to 65% of dieters return to their pre-dieting weight before the 3 year mark. That's according to *Gary Foster, Ph.D.*, Director of the Eating Disorder Program at the University of Pennsylvania.

The Ketogenic Diet can be used for successful rapid weight loss when used properly. And THOUSANDS of people report up to a pound a day lost!

This is an introductory take-action guide for understanding and using the Ketogenic Diet to lose weight fast and effectively. It will give you a huge advantage in forcing your body to lose fat and keep it off for life!

Nutrition and fitness professionals around the globe recommend healthy dietary changes and regular exercise to lose weight permanently. This is where the Ketogenic Diet comes in. An eating strategy that's not about starving yourself. It's a scientifically proven diet to lose weight that actually forces your body to chemically alter the fuel your body normally uses for energy. With the Ketogenic low-carb eating style you force your body to maximize fat burn for energy and blast fat stores in the process.

Is the Ketogenic Diet safe?

The American Journal of Clinical Nutrition points out no species could have survived millions of years without natural periods where glucose wasn't available for energy burn. Scientists also point out that natural ketogenesis occurs when you are sleeping.

And because of the high-fat intake the Ketogenic Diet allows calories to be cut drastically without feeling deprived and hungry.

There are thousands of people eating Ketogenic style that have claimed to lose between 20 and 30 pounds in just one month! *The Ketogenic Diet Resource* has success stories with people happily losing 30 pounds in 30 days and going strong!

We are going to have a look at the Ketogenic Diet for weight loss and other natural health benefits, while outlining a sample eating plan, food list, and exercise tips to help you reach your weight loss goals quickly. **FAST** weight loss is the focus and this eating strategy can make it happen for **YOU**.

This guide teaches you all about the Ketogenic Diet basics and how you can use this fast weight loss eating plan to rejig your body to use fat stores for energy first, while guiding you step by step towards a healthier lifestyle.

Don't miss out on this guide that teaches you how to take control of your fat TODAY!